# Table of Contents

The Impact of Alcohol Consumption on People with Epilepsy

# Alcohol Induced Epilepsy Seizures: Risks and Recommendations

# 1. Introduction

This essay will focus on the primary toxic factor of alcohol and epileptic parts previously shown for alcohol-induced strokes. In addition, to avert the continuation of early alcohol-induced epilepsy seizures, the essay will highlight new management strategies and specialists with alcohol use and non-use disorders. Special attention will be on necessary techniques of treatment alterations and drugs, illness evaluation techniques, and continuing tendencies of early episodes of epilepsy induced by alcohol. However, epilepsy has been associated with loss of awareness, and it is because of a reduction in movement or behavior that occurs in 60 seconds or less, before or after general convulsions for approximately 30 minutes. Management-free patients have practical and psychiatric antiepileptic medicines (AEDs). Etiology is inadequate, with a relationship between the underhanded application and epilepsy. Alcohol has an essential power in developing new epilepsy and ending etiology.

An epilepsy seizure is a sudden occurrence of involuntary muscular spasms or convulsions. It happens to epilepsy patients. We know that there are many factors that can induce seizures in epilepsy patients. One out of ten people have an episode induced by excessive drinking. After the first stroke, exceeding the blood treatment of toxic concentrations of alcohol (BAC of 0.08% or more) may make these consequences more severe and vary the way an individual feels. Alcohol-induced strokes can last up to

24 hours and can include enduring hospitalization as well as premature health difficulties. In general, patients who manage severe alcohol withdrawal have better consequences than those who experience seizures on their bloodstream or before the intense withdrawal of alcohol.

## 2. Understanding Epilepsy and Seizures

Not all seizures are the same. There are many kinds of seizures, some once associated with epilepsy, some not. Some seizures strike in plain view, like tonic clonic seizures that can cause convulsions and result in the person falling down and jerking uncontrollably. Other seizures are harder to detect, like absence, or petit mal seizures, which are associated with staring off. These are more subtle and may appear as daydream-like states. Epilepsy is a family of related disorders with one or more types of seizures.

A seizure is a sudden surge of electrical activity in the brain. A person who has two or more unprovoked seizures is considered to have epilepsy. The brain controls the body with a range of 'electrical' signals. That is what we see when a heart beats or a complex set of muscles participate in complex movements. Normally, those billions of signals all fall into place just as the most complex mechanisms in the universe course and we go about our business as usual...even if that business is enduring a fortune of relative good fortune or bad. A seizure happens when now and again many signs approach a "resolution" at the same time and the brain cannot keep track of all the traffic. It's more like a computer crash, one where macros all get involved in a mechanical dance and frontal lobes or corpus callosum just gives up on the reporting-in process.

Epilepsy is a neurological disorder characterized by recurrent, unprovoked seizures. Best estimates suggest at least three million Americans live with the condition. But, of the 60 million people worldwide diagnosed with epilepsy, too many are managed inappropriately, inequitably, or not at all. One size does not fit all, and understanding each person's unique condition is the necessary first step in delivering effective treatment.

## 2. Understanding Epilepsy and Seizures

Not all seizures are the same. There are many kinds of seizures, some once associated with epilepsy, some not. Some seizures strike in plain view, like tonic clonic seizures that can cause convulsions and result in the person falling down and jerking uncontrollably. Other seizures are harder to detect, like absence, or petit mal seizures, which are associated with staring off. These are more subtle and may appear as daydream-like states. Epilepsy is a family of related disorders with one or more types of seizures.

A seizure is a sudden surge of electrical activity in the brain. A person who has two or more unprovoked seizures is considered to have epilepsy. The brain controls the body with a range of 'electrical' signals. That is what we see when a heart beats or a complex set of muscles participate in complex movements. Normally, those billions of signals all fall into place just as the most complex mechanisms in the universe course and we go about our business as usual...even if that business is enduring a fortune of relative good fortune or bad. A seizure happens when now and again many signs approach a "resolution" at the same time and the brain cannot keep track of all the traffic. It's more like a computer crash, one where macros all get involved in a mechanical dance and frontal lobes or corpus callosum just gives up on the reporting-in process.

Epilepsy is a neurological disorder characterized by recurrent, unprovoked seizures. Best estimates suggest at least three million Americans live with the condition. But, of the 60 million people worldwide diagnosed with epilepsy, too many are managed inappropriately, inequitably, or not at all. One size does not fit all, and understanding each person's unique condition is the necessary first step in delivering effective treatment.

## 2.1. Epilepsy Basics

Two broad categories of epilepsy diagnoses are focal and generalized seizures. Focal seizures affect restricted parts of the brain that can disrupt particular behavior or movements. Then, this category determines if an individual may also experience focal to bilateral tonic-clonic seizures (formerly known as grand mal). Bilateral tonic-clonic seizures provoke a loss of consciousness and affect the whole part of both brain hemispheres. Focal seizures, by contrast, only clear the two-part cerebral hemispheres of this phenomenon. Idiopathic generalizing seizures occur in the brain of those with a normal condition (normal MRI or anger). These seizures are also known as 'petit mal' or 'absence' of short, general brain malfunction. Symptomatic generalized seizures are those recurrent by brain disorders, such as brain damage or brain blood vessels. Drug-resistant epilepsy, which is inadequate to alleviate with conduction drugs, is refractory. Ultimately, we endure the overall stress of an environment that may boost the frequency of a seizure. Alcohol consumption is a main trigger for many people with epilepsy, especially those who binge drink. Demonstrated was a link that pints are enough to fire an epileptic alcohol-induced crisis. Epileptics should be cautioned about this and be reasonably stressed amine from alcohol.

Epilepsy is a neurological disorder of the brain that affects approximately 0.5-1% of the world's population. With more than 180,000 new cases reported each year in the United States, an overall estimated 3 million individuals nationwide are currently living with epilepsy and experience seizures. This condition presents with seizures, unprovoked physical or behavioral convulsions due to fluctuating convoluted activities of nerve cells. One seizure doesn't mean an individual has epilepsy, but recurrences are necessary for accurate diagnosis. Psychosocial problems, loss of developmental, occupational, and regulators may occur in cases of continued seizures as a result. Prevention regimens of seizures vary according to an individual's type and degree of severity. Antiepileptic medications are a common course of treatment, along with counseling and education to comprehensive epilepsy care centers. Unfortunately for some, seizures may remain uncontrolled and turn into alcohol-related seizures through alcoholism and excessive drinking.

8. Focal seizures with dyscognitive (complex partial) features Such seizures begin as focal seizures in one brain area, but impair memory and awareness and can affect consciousness. In some cases, people retain awareness but find they are unable to communicate or are 'locked out' of speech.

7. Akinetic seizures Muscles lose their tone, causing sudden falls and injuries to occur. Unusual forms of fitting that have also been encountered in people with epilepsy include:

6. Clonic seizures These seizures cause muscles to jerk rhythmically and are less likely to happen in adults. They can also involve sudden falls and therefore injuries.

5. Tonic seizures Such seizures completely involve the entire brain, with the muscles producing increased tone to create a stiff posture. They could result in falls and injuries. Muscles such as the neck and back may also become tight causing arching movements. These seizures can occur during sleep, with possible resultant bedwetting and can also present as nighttime or nocturnal attacks with injuries.

4. Tonic-clonic seizures or generalized seizures Such seizures affect the whole brain from the outset. Great force affects all joints and breathing may be affected causing 'pallor' or occasionally a bluish color of the lips and mouth.

3. Motor seizures These seizures are divided into two main types according to the initial symptoms that are entirely distinctive.

2. Absence seizures Also previously known as petit mal, these types affect children aged from 4 years to adolescence. The person having the seizure appears to be 'absent' and is likely to have no memory of the seizure afterward. Emotionally common triggers include feeling stressed or if excited.

1. Focal seizures These forms mean that the seizures are focal, which indicates that they initiate in one region of the brain. Partial seizures can also exhibit automatisms, whereby simple, repetitive movements including lip smacking, buttoning and unbuttoning clothes, scratching or gestures, such as picking at things in the air or trying to pick items off your clothing, may occur.

# 3. Alcohol Consumption and Epilepsy

To understand how alcohol provokes seizures, one should know what effects alcohol has on the brain. Alcohol modulates the activity of several neurotransmitters in the brain. For example, it inhibits glutamatergic activity while enhancing the activity of the inhibitory GABA_A receptor. When alcohol levels accumulate to toxic levels, it might antagonize mechanisms of the GABA receptor, which causes the compromised inhibitory action of the neurotransmitter GABA and reduces synaptic GABA. Subsequently, the excessive excitatory neurotransmitter glutamate gets released. During chronic periods of diminished synaptic bases of GABA-A activations, the neurons within the brain tend to be more excitatory than inhibitory. Withdrawal from alcohol exposure would approximate the lower limit for excitation in an environment surrounded by abnormal inhibitory cells. When people are in this vulnerable state, the supposedly hyper-excited neurons discharge synchronously, leading to seizure activity.

Epilepsy is a neurological condition that affects the functioning of the nervous and motor systems. It is characterized by recurrent episodes of convulsions, sensory disturbances, abnormal behavior, loss of consciousness, or unresponsiveness. However, the seizures caused by epilepsy may be induced by many other factors alongside the neurological condition. Alcohol, for instance, might become a trigger of seizures if the individual is prone to having a seizure. Additionally, one may develop alcohol-induced epilepsy after being chronically exposed to alcohol during periods of heavy drinking. The intoxicating factor of alcohol might provoke ambiguous brain activity, once suddenly removed, which causes a class of generalized seizures called alcohol withdrawal seizures (AWS).

## 3.1. Effects of Alcohol on the Brain

Epilepsy is a condition of the brain not functioning properly due to abnormal cortical activity, which manifests in seizures. The root cause of epilepsy is still debatable, but there are a plethora of known errors such as genetic mutations, trauma, infectious diseases, brain damage, and prenatal injury. The nervous system contains a balance between excitatory neurotransmitters and inhibitory. While it is possible for a seizure to occur from excessive alcohol intake or withdrawal with an individual without epilepsy, long-term alcohol dependency or acute withdrawal can exacerbate epileptic activity in those with epilepsy. In some cases of long-term alcoholism, those who do not have epilepsy can still develop an epilepsy disorder with thiamine deficiency being a likely factor, Wernicke's encephalopathy, as well as Korsakoff's syndrome, which is a memory disorder.

The impact of alcohol on the brain is substantial. Alcohol exhibits a variety of properties that can affect the brain system. Alcohol is a "downer" or depressant that hinders cognitive functions such as inhibitions, which can cause an individual to make risky decisions, speech, and balance, to name a few. Many experience the release of the naturally occurring chemical and neurotransmitter, dopamine, as a surge of reward from participating in certain activities, for example, rock climbing. In fact, anytime we engage in some activity, our brain creates a "pleasure pathway." Drugs such as alcohol greatly increase the release of dopamine and double that time. The primary neurotransmitter involved in epileptic occurrence is γ-aminobutyric acid (GABA). Ethanol functions as a sedative by facilitating GABA through the GABA-A receptor channel and hyperpolarizing neurons. Alcohol decreases cellular excitability and synaptic transmission of neurons in the brain by increasing the influx of chloride (Cl-) ions. The mechanism by which ethanol increases the influx of these Cl- ions is through the agonist binding of GABA.

## 3.2. Alcohol Induced Seizures

Therefore, to effectively manage someone presenting with epilepsy accompanied by frequent alcohol consumption, the physician not only needs to be aware of alcohol-induced seizures and the risk of precipitating SE but also be able to distinguish between other potential neurodevelopmental effects on brain function by personal alcohol use, which can be considerably significant (Box 2). Evidence suggests effects of chronic alcohol exposure on neurotransmitter systems, oxidative stress, and excessive release of glutamate from upregulated NMDA receptors. Ion channels and membrane-bound neurotransmitter transport systems are also dysregulated when a patient accustomed to large amounts of alcohol suffers alcohol withdrawal. Also, glutathione concentrations decrease for up to three years post-drinking cessation.

In the United States, alcohol withdrawal has long been recognized as a primary risk factor for the development of seizures and epilepsy. Laying the groundwork for the epidemic of alcohol obtained among patents has unique seizure risk. The kindling effect, first documented in 1984 by Graham Goddard, is used to justify this connection between alcohol acquisition from withdrawal seizure to-induced acute vocal-appearing natural history epileptic seizures and post-traumatic epilepsy. It is a neuroplastic phenomenon from recurrent sub-threshold (e.g., withdrawal) epileptic seizures, or ictal-like physiological changes, that increases seizure susceptibility. Although de novo status epilepticus (SE) obtained during an episode of binge drinking should be approached parsimoniously until proven otherwise, as a general rule, an individual drinking large amounts of alcohol for the first time the most superimposable responses and side effects using dynamic dose-response. If previously obtained a single time-limited seizure, day or so after the last drink, lasting less than 2–3 min.

# 4. Risk Factors for Alcohol Induced Seizures

The American Academy of Neurology could show that alcoholism, i.e. the daily intake of large amounts of alcohol (more than 4 ounces of pure alcohol), increases the risk of seizure occurrence. In studies on the consumption habits typical for the country, it is frequently discussed whether the frequency or the amount of intake is the most important contributing factor to the occurrence of seizures (epileptic, unprovoked) or also AIS. Whether either playing the frequency of intake or the amount has led to the seizures is a question which is still unclear. While in principle all authors consider these factors central, Waberski and Elger state that recent information supports the higher relevance of the amount of alcohol intake, being close to known: the more has been taken in during a given time (hours in most studies), the more seizures. Generally speaking, seizure occurrence may be explained by the underlying electrical neurological 'hyperactivity in the human brain. While it is well accepted that AIS might lower the convulsive threshold, the exact pathophysiological mechanisms underlying seizures in AIS are still not well understood.

Alcohol-induced seizures (AIS) are a risk factor, especially for individuals with epilepsy. Nevertheless, not every person who drinks alcohol and suffers from epilepsy has an alcohol-induced seizure. Several risk factors contributing to the likelihood of suffering AIS are known as personal and alcohol consumption factors. It is clearly shown that the frequency, as well as the amount of alcohol intake, influence tolerance as well as the frequency of seizures occurring in epilepsy. However, factors like type, gender, and age of the affected person have to be considered.

## 4.1. Individual Susceptibility

Some US-based denominational AA elders unceasingly demonstrate that the numbers of poor who become 'spiritual' or 'religious' as their last resort approach the ratios of general religious distribution known from the 19th century. For example, 2% Muslims, 35% Christians, with 50% Catholics and 10% Jews, herding in the villages of Russia, say, immediately after the killing lifetime was concluded and while there was no KGB to play some part. Gathered with the maximum participative assistance of successive pronoun referring, they sounded even Policemanish at those moments. Their membership (love?) rivals such pinnacle political ideologies as fascism, communism, and radical empiricism. Their publication circulation rivals the bibles—all bibles, as their potential alcoholics are altering, with that Gideon's gimmick for courtrooms, the literal Olde Tyme Masculine Noun Gone. They have grown to 60% men, from what once were barely half that. Hard-heartedness might start like this too. They have a celebrity pool, a voter turnout, and a new (2002) journal, etc., and no fewer than forty-four U.S. commercial real-estate storefronts in every major metropolitan demographic distribution.

The discovery of a large variation in the pattern of alcohol consumption between individuals has brought the field of individual differences research into focus. Individual drinking patterns can be conditioned by various health or environmental factors. Human genetic research has shown that interindividual variations may further be based on a genetic susceptibility to develop alcohol dependence. In a similar way, the sensitivity to alcohol of central regulators, the heightened reward, or the development of tolerance to the toxic brain exposure may explain why some drinkers can consume large amounts of alcohol over many years and remain free of seizures, whereas others, even with minimal exposure, are susceptible to alcohol-induced seizures. As there may be strong and specific individual susceptibility factors that make certain patients more vulnerable to epilepsy provoked by liquor, there may be differential sensitivities concerning the risks and benefits of alcohol consumption within the broad population of AE patients. This would then call for risk estimates for individual patients. In any case, these considerations pave the way to individual care with regard to the risk of alcohol-induced seizures in epilepsy.

## 4.2. Frequency and Amount of Alcohol Consumption

5.2. Abstinence and Change of Alcohol Consumption The probability of gene polymorphisms to no longer use newly produced GABA or to change with ADF (alcohol dehydrogenase) as compliance rate is not known and therefore to be used. Such subjects are excellent candidates for future test fusions. Statistically, at least one quarter of alcohol-drinking subjects are unlikely to change their amount, a phenomenon described as autodemission.

Quantitative aspects concerning alcohol drinking patterns may be decisive for the development of alcohol-induced epilepsy seizures. At the beginning of the 20th century, Fischer and Carel indicated that more than 30 g of alcohol resulted in vitarum incrementum, which is an epicritic surmenage, but inappetentitus resulted from consumption exceeding 70 g/day. In a telephone survey to characterize the implication of alcohol poisoning in epileptic individuals, Høgset et al. summarized 240 subjects with epilepsy who stated that they decreased their alcohol use to about 2.9 g/day after a median time of 7 years after cancer disease. It is known that hazardous drinkers are more likely to reduce their alcohol consumption after myocardial infarction. The onset of epilepsy in PWE (people with epilepsy) may be of particular concern, even more remarkable, which, if applicable, may lead to the development of meaningful preventive strategies. Future recommendations now help to predict the severity of alcohol withdrawal in epilepsy and will allow for an evidence-based strategy to reduce the risk of associated seizures.

# 5. Management and Prevention Strategies

Nonpharmacologic strategies, like adherence programs and lifestyle changes, must be pursued minimally to diminish the risk and impact of seizures. Compliance with prescribed medical treatment and lifestyle modifications holds great potential in treating seizure control. There is a direct connection between inconsistencies in medication use and the occurrence of seizures. Strategies for increasing compliance include implementing education on the importance of regular medication use and treatment cure; designation of reminder systems, such as pillboxes and phones with alarm capabilities; provision of home-based support, such as trained professionals, to supplement patient adherence; and formulation of electronic medical records for rapid and accurate recording of adherence difficulties for relevant care providers. Seizure plans can be established and are beneficial for people at increased risk of seizure with lower thresholds such as struggling to find a correct medication and dose or not having good control of their seizures or who experiences breakthrough seizures. These can often be devised by your primary care doctor and can also help to guide work, activity, and more to avoid any consequences of a provoked seizure.

Management and prevention strategies. There are two different focal points for managing alcohol-related concerns. The first plan is to assess and guide in reducing the risk of alcohol-provoked seizures while steadily assessing the overall health of that individual and providing care and direction to maintain quality of life outside of the home. At the same time, providers can help provide information and guidance on drug interactions and ways to make your medications less reactive to alcohol. The second plan is to drastically lower the amount of alcohol to ease up stress on the body itself, causing fewer seizures, bedwetting, or a headache. With this plan, our team would also like to evaluate and risk-stratify the presumptive patient with epilepsy or seizures looking for who is at an increased risk of alcohol-related injury and should not be discharged. A shift in priorities towards systems-based strategies to prevent missteps in the prehospital, initial evaluation, inpatient management, and discharge planning will help save more lives from immediate risks of seizures.

## 5.1. Medication Adherence

Clinicians address alcohol consumption as well as encourage abstinence or safe limits for a variety of interventions for PWE. Approaches may include motivational interviewing, alcohol management counseling, written materials that reinforce safe drinking advisements or abstinence, or review of the association of alcohol and seizures. Physicians should recognize that excessive alcohol use can lead to poor medication adherence. In the case of AIE, non-adherent individuals who take AEDs provide an additional part of the population who may be at risk for seizures unrelated to medication withdrawal. Despite the importance of medication management, few guidelines regarding AIE and alcohol consumption are available.

Achieving seizure control in people with epilepsy (PWE) typically involves medication adherence and management. Adherence to taking AEDs can be an issue for adults with newly diagnosed epilepsy, as an epilepsy diagnosis can alter an individual's psychological, social, and emotional functioning. It is unknown whether young adults are more susceptible to medication non-adherence due to an increased risk for unresolved neurodevelopmental issues. For individuals with psychogenic non-epileptic seizures (PNES), the influence of medications on seizure frequency is also an adjuvant mechanism.

## 5.2. Lifestyle Modifications

According to recently updated guidelines by the American College of Physicians, behavioral things someone might engage in, including managing stress, practicing yoga, and walking or getting moderate exercise, can be just as beneficial as medication in preventing future low-back pain. Someone engaging in lifestyle modifications (in addition to prescribed anti-epileptic medication) will likely: 1) feel like they are engaging in positive activities to help themselves (an increased sense of self-efficacy), 2) improve their overall well-being (not just their physical health), 3) feel in control of all life situations (i.e., "I don't want to feel like my world is constantly going to end if something potentially bad ever happens." Such control is known as "sense of coherence," and is impacted by the ability to make good decisions), and 4) have a lowered risk of alcohol-induced seizures because they are either not drinking or are drinking in moderation in conjunction with environmental and personal factors that aren't conducive to seizures.

Lifestyle factors might be just as important when it comes to protecting against alcohol-induced seizures. In comparison to a normative sample, adults with epilepsy engage in fewer healthy lifestyle behaviors. Healthier individuals often report fewer problems overall in memory and non-memory domains, and respond better to treatment than those living an unhealthier lifestyle. Such findings may suggest that developing healthier lifestyles could be a potentially useful avenue to explore in terms of alcohol-induced seizures in PWE.

# 6. Recommendations for Individuals with Epilepsy

Have you read these facts and wondered: is this safe? What are the implications of this guidance for me, or for people who have epilepsy? If you have epilepsy and are interested in medicine, then you will know that guidelines are made according to the best evidence available from a group of people who have similar conditions. In this case, the evidence tells us that many safeguards should be in place when providing advice to not only people in the community but also (especially) to those who have epilepsy. In addition, any recommendations should be personalized, as different individuals have different needs, risk factors, and medical conditions. Unfortunately, we know that many people living with epilepsy have never even heard this simplified risk profile and many more have not had the opportunity to think about the implications of alcohol intake for their seizures. In order to facilitate self-management, generic guidelines must be translated into meaningful advice for each individual.

- Adults should limit their intake to no more than two standard drinks on any day to reduce the risk of injury from alcohol. - If you do not consume alcohol, do not start. - If you are unsure about your drinking patterns, consider seeking advice from a health professional. - Always take your anti-seizure medication as directed by your doctor. - Be aware of the effects of alcohol on your seizure threshold. - Have regular check-ups to monitor your epilepsy and any drinking problems. - There is no safe level of alcohol during pregnancy or when trying for pregnancy. - If you have drunk alcohol before you knew you were pregnant, discuss this with your doctor. - Speak to your doctor if you are worried about your alcohol use or if alcohol is placing you at risk of injury.

## 6.1. Safe Alcohol Consumption Guidelines

Based on the evidence from preclinical and clinical studies, we provide safe drinking guideline recommendations for people with epilepsy to prevent alcohol-induced seizures. These guideline recommendations describe the short-term and long-term impact and risks of alcohol; how people with current and previous drinking problems have a more significant chance of both short-term and long-term alcohol-associated risk; practical applications; relevant pharmacological aspects of alcohol consumption in people with epilepsy, including improving mood and antiepileptic drug concentrations.

Not drinking alcohol is the safest option for people with epilepsy who have a higher risk of seizures. However, the decision to drink alcohol is an individual decision and a person's attitudes, beliefs, and lifestyle are influential. The risks associated with increased seizure frequency are influenced by the amount of alcohol and pattern of drinking. For some people, only small amounts of alcohol or only on separate occasions could be sufficient to increase their risk of seizures. Cross-sectional population-based surveys have indicated that more people with epilepsy were drinking more than the recommended weekly intake guidelines compared to those without epilepsy. One approach is to provide people with individualized recommendations based on their risk of seizures and pattern in drinking. However, little is known about the association between alcohol consumption, prevention advice, motor vehicle accidents, or injuries for people with epilepsy. In this recommendation statement, we provide safe drinking guideline recommendations from expert opinion with practical applications adapted from national drinking guideline recommendations.

Safe alcohol consumption guidelines.

## 6.2. Seeking Professional Help

- Get into a routine of regular GP visits and any other important healthcare appointments if possible. Suggested topics to discuss to help reduce the impact of problems: - Challenging seizure times (such as early morning or in public). - Monitoring of any side effects of treatment or epilepsy impact. - Concerns regarding seizure control changes, impact of seizures or aura on daily living. - Professionals in this area could discuss (on their routine visits) with people: - Work, training or education, diet and exercise, issues from your latest blood tests and seizure, and treatment diaries and understanding of epilepsy. - Other treatments and issues should be discussed with a neurology specialist or contact if problems.

People with epilepsy are encouraged to drink alcohol responsibly and within the recommended safe limits. Many people may seek the guidance of a neurology specialist, such as a neurologist or epilepsy specialist nurse, to best understand and discuss their personal risk associated with drinking. This will be beneficial for those with alcohol-related seizures, or who notice increased seizures in connection with their drinking. People with epilepsy of any severity should consult their healthcare professional if they have alcohol-related concerns. This will help to ensure any specialist healthcare professional supports you or those close to you in being able to find solutions to challenging issues. This may help you to avoid high alcohol-related epilepsy-related risks. Raised awareness of increased risk behaviour can be shared with those around you as part of the support network, including family and friends.

# 7. Support Systems and Resources

There are certain risks associated with alcohol in epilepsy. This is especially true when first diagnosed or changes are made in medications. Overconsumption of alcohol or the inappropriate time or amount of consumption can cause isolated seizures. Alcohol-induced seizures are those leading to status epilepticus that can lead to epilepsy, are less severe than that, and are characterized as alcohol-related. The threat of an alcoholic drink lowering the seizure threshold where attacks may be triggered is not the only difficulty associated with alcohol and epilepsy. In fact, the opposite is true: the risk of severe liver damage over medications taken in the long term; the possibility of overlooking the required amount of medications; and the low spirits and low energies frequently associated with the return of alcohol again, all raise several other genuine questions. Some individuals with epilepsy, though, appear to be able to handle moderate quantities of alcohol quite safely. In moderation, most people can drink alcohol and have seizures, so long as their illness is well treated and, significantly, well regulated.

When you're diagnosed with epilepsy, it's important to have a support system. Family and friends can provide the necessary support as your body and lifestyle change. It's important that the trust and understanding between you and those who care for you are well-established. Counselling is often a recommendation for people with epilepsy. This may include sessions on an individual level, or you can join groups. Epilepsy Support Groups are found throughout the UK and worldwide, and can be an invaluable resource. It doesn't matter if you don't have epilepsy yourself, because both people with epilepsy and their families are welcome to attend these meetings. You may find that you have a lot in common with other people who have had the same conditions. Rely on each other for support, share your experiences, and possibly learn from one another. If you have not already done so, please use the Epilepsy Action App to look for an assistance group near you.

## 7.1. Family and Friends

This is a time when an epilepsy specialist can, jointly with the consumer, share in the development of the reduced-risk harm minimization approach. When talking with the consumer, the epilepsy specialist can motivate the consumer to feel the joy and benefits of arousal and alcohol, rather than abstinence.

Preventive discussions have to be supported with an understanding of the needs of the person with epilepsy for social contact, the opportunities to develop personal, educational, and employment skills, and to ensure an enjoyable life. Sporting, musical, or artistic talents can be greatest when at one time alcohol consumption is experienced. To reduce the risk of seizures occurring, alcohol should not be consumed in times of excess drinking. Only where the consumer has observed and knows that there is a low risk of seizures is it safe for them to extend the range of drinks taken in a single night, or in a moment of "binge- or spree-drinking" have small sips of a range of alcoholic beverages.

The family plays a central role in providing and receiving help in living with epilepsy. For some people with epilepsy, the greatest extent of stigmatization and misunderstanding is found within the family where the secrecy can present a particular challenge. The relative chances of living with fear and impairment of a social life, or school and work opportunities, are increased where a person with epilepsy experiences seizures after some heavy drinking. Families often appreciate the chance of meeting with a professional, including social workers or clinical nurse specialists, to talk openly about the long- and short-term risks. The same is true with friends of a person who has demonstrated tolerance to alcohol-induced seizures; the opportunities to seek advice may maintain health and living conditions.

## 7.2. Support Groups

Staff at these organizations can provide you with the name and phone number of the contact person in your area. The more than 410 support groups in the directory consistently provide a support and information-giving function. Some are designed to deal with groups of people based on certain medical conditions such as asthma or epilepsy. Although being operated by enABKCH, epilepsy support groups in particular are strongly linked with particular communities within metropolitan, outer-metropolitan, and rural areas to embrace the unique experiences of living with epilepsy. Epilepsy can present unique challenges because it's likely to be largely hidden from friends by family who don't understand their experience or the stigma attached to people living with epilepsy in their community. For people living with epilepsy, support groups can provide a safe, empathetic environment where they are accepted and people understand. Unfortunately, for some, it is the only part of their life where they feel this way. Support groups often have guest speakers to provide information or leave resources for group members at meetings to take away. In particular, a large portion of the group-specific website resources for each support group link has been some support groups providing information for the support person, not just the person living with epilepsy. The references given in these support groups are written by the Epilepsy Foundation. Apart from that, many groups are capable of providing information in languages other than English.

Epilepsy is not welcome; however, an exception is made for college-aged friends of members of the group not living with epilepsy who are interested in learning more about the condition. The visitor center is for those new to the world of epilepsy. Often, people living with epilepsy after a new diagnosis can find life very challenging. The issues associated with the need to integrate medical appointments, medication, low self-esteem, educational barriers, and many other hurdles can make even simple life activities difficult. Being able to speak to others who are living with epilepsy and can share similar experiences in a supportive and confidential environment can provide the knowledge that difficulties can be overcome.

There are organizations in Australia that can put you in touch with a support group in your area. Support groups can offer you support, unconditional acceptance, understanding, and encouragement for all your efforts. They will also offer information in the form of fact sheets, newsletters, and occasional invited guests from areas of interest such as medication, surgery, and stress management. Support group meetings are confidential. The only exceptions are where some members of the group plan visits to hospitals or information nights, in which case the permission of the hospital is sought first, and some visitor centers and group conferences are also open to staff and students of the Epilepsy Unit, but only where the patients and their carers agree to it.

# 8. Public Health Implications

An updated report on the costs and unmet needs of epilepsy in the United States has been developed and includes societal costs from an additional set of recommendations and increasing access to specialty care. However, neither contained the concerns of those with alcohol-induced epilepsy seizures. This is not just a circuit of addiction concern and warrants a public health response that the specialist needs to acknowledge. Concerted actions to reduce risk during consumption cannot necessarily lead to a reduction in seizures for those who have a non-specific seizure threshold. The spectrum of what can be recommended to reduce risk or rescue from harm during a seizure with alcohol is vast and probably more than any one news source could capture. However, if these concerns can root into actions and interventions, we can begin to follow trends of change in 5 years nationally for those who fear an addressable public health harm.

5.5 million Americans have had an alcohol-induced epileptic seizure in their lifetime. More than 85% of those reporting a history of alcohol-induced epileptic seizures met criteria for an alcohol use disorder at some point in their lives. These individuals are also at an earlier age of onset of epilepsy compared to those with epilepsy alone. The burden of those who have died in association with an alcohol-induced epileptic seizure contributed to a loss of life of 4658 years due to premature mortality, which was higher for females than males. This public health concern leads to the use of approximately 1% of the yearly costs allocated to the participants in the National Health and Nutrition Examination Surveys 20015–2016.

## 9. Future Research Directions

In summary, there are now hypotheses that warrant focused attention, which have developed from new data and new analytic techniques. Other areas in need of attention include the most basic and dose-dependent aspects of ethanol neuropharmacology on seizure threshold, replication and integration of current data, and newly imagined areas such as non-animal model systems. Such feasibility and proof-of-concept studies could contribute new mechanisms for future translational study. Protective factors such as abstinence and chronic administration of supportive compounds warrant investigation. Finally, methodological innovation and expansion are needed to continue to quantify the boundaries of neurotoxicity. It is our hope that with potential new directions, providers will have increasingly robust information that will be used to provide the most optimal guidance to those who have sustained a potential alcohol withdrawal seizure.

At its juncture of development, focused basic and applied research can lead to new discoveries that can influence treatment standards for alcohol-induced seizures. It is hoped that practice and policy can be informed by the evolving research. A variety of areas are in need of further experimentation, meta-analysis (or re-analysis), or methodological development.

# 10. Conclusion

Numerous reports from clinical, epidemiological, and experimental studies around the globe are solid testimonial reflecting a high prevalence of seizures associated with alcoholism. AEDs should be usually avoided if the benefit of use in a patient is lower than the adverse effect. If the history is unclear, it is pragmatic to initiate AEDs as the investigation takes form. All patients with epilepsy are at a risk of developing a seizure if they are intoxicated or their AED is reduced prematurely. The use of AEDs should be cautiously documented and should be pursued judiciously, especially while taking alcohol history. The alcohol withdrawal seizures should be ideally treated with benzodiazepines and, if required, with anticonvulsants. Status epilepticus should be promptly identified and treated. The chronic treatment, overall, requires comprehensive care with cognitive and behavioral therapies and the prescription of AEDs wherever it is indicated. Hyperexcitability with neuronal connections and networks could be manifest directly leading to kindling due to the same zone or leading to the secondary generalization. Kinder May Last Lifetime, Once Kindled. Even a single seizure does not mean the person is handling epilepsy. Therefore, with regard to driving and participation in adventure and risky activities, a prudent approach with counseling and education is of great importance.

Alcohol-induced seizures in people who have compromised brain tissue are an intriguing occurrence. It is noteworthy that the biotransformation of alcohol into an excitatory metabolite, acetaldehyde, in the brain, along with alterations of the glutamatergic and GABAergic systems, makes this study pertinent in the future management of AIEs, especially in PWEs. This premise indicates the necessity of a corroborating randomized controlled trial with learned safety measures. Alcohol use has been reported to contribute to a significant increase in the prevalence of seizures and epilepsy in resource-poor countries. The natural progression of alcohol misusing patients to epilepsy is evident in the relationship of one problem to the other. The dose and the duration of alcohol misuse play a critical role. The research in the field does hint that alcohol induces its own kind of epilepsy, which might differ from the one not related to alcohol.

# The Impact of Alcohol Consumption on People with Epilepsy

# 1. Introduction to Epilepsy and Seizures

- Forgetting to take medications or not taking them regularly - Physical tiredness - Certain foods or specific food additives or sensitivities - Alcohol or drug withdrawal - Dehydration - Hormonal changes, particularly the changing hormone levels during a woman's menstrual cycle - Staying up very late and lack of sleep - Illness - Fever - Stress - Flashing lights - Extreme heat and cold - Injury/trauma.

The factors that people with epilepsy have reported to trigger their seizures include:

Focal (formerly called partial) seizures are feelings of abnormal sensations or perhaps jerking movements. These seizures are typically localized to a part of one brain hemisphere. Focal seizures may proceed to a bilateral seizure which affects both sides of the brain and the person's behavior and consciousness.

Generalized seizures affect both sides of the brain and also the person with epilepsy's behavior and consciousness.

A seizure is a brief episode of symptoms due to abnormal or excessive electrical discharge in the brain. Seizures vary from very short and nearly undetectable to long periods of vigorous shaking or physical collapse. A person is diagnosed with epilepsy when they have had two or more seizures. Catamenial epilepsy is a type of epilepsy that is linked to a woman's menstrual cycle and is associated with two main types of seizures - generalized and focal seizures.

# Epilepsy and Seizures

## 1.1. Definition and Types of Epilepsy

Epilepsy is classified by type, location on the brain, effects, and can also be of unclassifiable type. Partial seizures occur when only a part of the brain experiences an electrical surge. Based on the mode of spread of electrical surge, partial seizures are of two categories: simple partial seizures and complex partial seizures. Generalized seizures simultaneously send abnormal electrical discharges throughout the entire brain. Generalized epilepsy is complex and divided than partial epilepsy consisting of various types of seizures occurring in any combination, each having a name, such as Absence seizures (formerly known as petit mal seizures), Myoclonic seizures, Tonic-clonic seizures—also called generalized tonic-clonic seizures and used to be known as grand mal seizures—, Tonic seizures, Clonic seizures, Atonic seizures. Status epilepticus is a life-threatening medical emergency in which seizures last for more than five minutes, or one seizure quickly follows another without allowing the patient to recover and consciousness to return.

Epilepsy is a disorder of the brain characterized by repeated seizures or fits, in which groups of cells in the brain send abnormal electrical signals. Seizures result in a wide range of symptoms, including loss of consciousness, episodes of blank staring, or repetitive movements such as chewing or hand rubbing. Imbalance of neurotransmitters, structural brain abnormalities, a family history of epilepsy, low birth weight, premature birth, or oxygen deprivation to the brain at birth have been identified as risk factors for epilepsy. Numerous types of seizures occur in epilepsy, and a physician will use a variety of methods, such as a seizure diary, electroencephalogram, magnetic resonance imaging, computed tomography, or blood tests, to diagnose them. Epilepsy can affect any person of any age, but it is more common in people aged 70 to 79 years. An estimated 50-60 million people worldwide have epilepsy.

## 1.2. Common Triggers for Seizures

It is important to note that there are other factors that may be specific to aetiologies of epilepsy rather than specific seizure types. For example, in patients with photosensitive epilepsy and individuals with learning disability and epilepsy, the content and duration of television exposure has been reported as a temporal lobe epilepsy in adults accompanied by intractable seizures. There is potential for a feedback loop to occur, where seizures wrought by alcohol withdrawal - be they relatively benign shakes or full-blown seizures - can promote further drinking by way of immediate, full-blown loss of control and urges to turn to alcohol. Thus, people with seizures may be encouraged to, in a sense, "test" each of these individual "ok" factors to see at what point their epilepsy crosses into "will make me have a seizure", particularly in those cases where alcohol consumption is driving epilepsy beyond what would naturally occur. This can lead to doubts as to what lifestyle changes are really safe and can ultimately convince people that their epilepsy can never be controlled, no matter what they do.

There are a wide variety of factors that can precipitate seizure activity, given that epilepsy alone forms such a complex group of syndromes. However, it is possible to linguistically characterise seizures according to specific triggers, for characterisation of the impact of an individual's lifestyle on their seizure susceptibility. Stress and tiredness are two of the most commonly reported triggers of most types of epilepsy and are associated with hormonal and neural changes. In Rolandic epilepsy (a localised form of epilepsy occurring in children) sleep deprivation is a typical seizure trigger, occurring on first arousal with a 'classical' morning pattern.

## 2. Understanding Alcohol Consumption

Alcohol is not digested in the stomach but absorbed in the intestine. Absorption is impaired in individuals with coeliac disease or those undergoing bypass surgery. Furthermore, individuals with epilepsy may be more prone to vomiting and thus have impaired absorption of alcohol. Individuals on multiple anti-epileptic medication have impaired hepatic CYP2E1 metabolism which is responsible for alcohol metabolism and will have a shift to alcohol elimination via the microsomal oxidase pathway in the brain, lung, and other extrahepatic tissues. The net result is likely to be higher levels of alcohol in the brain and other tissues, although more data is required to support this theory. Amounts of alcohol capable of increasing the time taken to reach peak drug levels (time to reach peak plasma concentration, Ttmax) and half-time (T1/2) would differ from the alcohol necessary to significantly increase maximum concentration (Cmax).

Drinking is often seen as part of the daily and social aspect of many lives. The actual number of people who drink alcohol in the UK is unknown due to unrecorded sources of the data; however, official statistics often suggest that Scottish individuals have higher alcohol consumption rates compared to the rest of the UK. As a result, the number of individuals belonging to one of the most common neurological disorders (epilepsy) having ingested alcohol is likely to be substantial. In normal healthy individuals, alcohol ingested is oxidised in the liver at a rate independent of alcohol concentration at a rate of 8g of ethanol/h which can liberate 7 kcal/g.

## 2.1. Metabolism of Alcohol in the Body

Alcohol has a rich history in human civilizations. It has been consumed for recreation, relaxation, rituals, medicinal purposes, as a drink of choice in some cultures, and even as a necessity in public health crises. However, it interacts with the neurological system of the body. Since epilepsy is also a neurological condition, it can be affected by alcohol consumption as well. Human cerebral blood flow studies have also shown a change in the regional cerebral blood flow control upon consumption of a small amount of alcohol daily. However, not most, but some studies have reported that patients with epilepsy increase drinking after the diagnosis of epilepsy. Like most populations, some individuals with epilepsy consume an excessive quantity of alcohol, indicating a drinking problem. Despite the consensus on an increased prevalence of epilepsy in alcohol drinkers, the underlying reason behind the latter's onset of seizures has not been clear in most of the studies conducted.

2.1. Alcohol is a chemical compound known as ethanol. It is a central nervous system depressant, meaning it slows down certain functions within the brain and the spinal cord. Alcohol cannot be stored in the body and must be metabolized or else it exerts toxic effects. Metabolism is the process by which the body breaks down and transforms a substance, sometimes making it possible to eliminate it from the body. It has been found that about 5-8% of the dose of alcohol consumed is eliminated through the lungs and kidneys. However, most alcohol metabolism occurs in the liver. This metabolic process is typically carried out in adults. It is slower in women than in men, mainly due to lower levels of water in the female body, and is slower still in elderly people. The body metabolizes alcohol following a zero-order kinetic pattern. That is, it metabolizes a constant amount of alcohol per unit time, regardless of the total amount of alcohol present.

## 2.2. Effects of Alcohol on the Brain

The National Institute on Alcoholism and Alcohol Abuse defines heavy drinking as consuming five or more drinks on a single occasion, with 25% of alcohol being of offense. Plus, two folks who drink hard have either intentions for good becoming a heavy drinker. Some factors may make folks with epilepsy more likely to have seizures related to alcohol, including real disabilities to afford affordability. Any seizures that may restore in any folks with either testimony and have either bronze rupts that go on almost a year after college. There are no easy answers for folks with epilepsy who want to drink altogether. Until more research is done, the risks and benefits of drinking should be discussed between you and the doctor.

The impact of alcohol consumption on people with epilepsy and marker candidates should be aware of the neurological effects of alcohol discussed in the following sections. The short-term and long-term effects of alcohol on the brain have been reviewed by Hyman et al. using functional magnetic resonance imaging and positron emission tomographic techniques. It has been suggested that alcohol affects the functions of neurotransmissions in the brain by inducing changes in the levels of several neurotransmitters and/or receptor activity. The brain and neurons are in the forms of a wide range of neurotransmitters; alcohol exerts its effects on neurotransmitter uptake, synthesis, release, or transmission. Based on its lipophilic properties, the functional effect of alcohol disrupts the integrity of the brain membrane, which in turn influences visions of the membrane-bound and cytoskeleton-associated proteins. There is damage due to chronic alcohol abuse that leads not only to brain atrophy but also white matter changes. Differences in genetics make some people more prone than others to developing intention, and further clinical evidence indicates that alcohol abuse results in neurological consequences. Some degree of neuroprotection is observed in the air of epilepsy and among people with normal cognition that begins.

## 3. Alcohol as a Seizure Trigger

It could be argued in favor of a certain cause and effect relationship, at least temporarily, between the consumption of alcohol and the occurrence of the seizure. In addition, it is known that those who continue to consume alcohol exacerbate their seizures, which decreases by suppressing the consumption of alcohol. However, curiously, daily alcohol intake discourages physical dependence on this substance and encourages dependence on antiepileptic drugs (AED). There is empirical evidence from studies that people who, on some occasions, have significantly increased blood alcohol levels have also increased rCBF for a few hours. Thus, this metabolic increase could be the cause of the seizure. Magnetoencephalography (MEG) and scalp EEG were unable to show the same similar phenomenon when alcohol was consumed, likely because these methods can only detect superficial activity and not deep EEG activity.

Although alcohol is known to be one of the main factors affecting seizures, only about 6% of people with epilepsy have alcohol as the only trigger. This would be related to the high dose consumed and/or the presence of addiction. People with epilepsy, particularly functional epilepsy, have a lower tolerance to alcohol than the general population concerning seizure triggers, such as sleep deprivation. They have a lower threshold for alcohol's threshold-lowering effect. Some factors that have made it possible to study the probability of alcohol affecting seizures are, on the one hand, the administration of a specific dose of alcohol to participants and, on the other hand, the possibility of random treatment and administration of a placebo to some of them.

## 3.1. Research Findings on Alcohol and Seizures

A review of independent population studies of the effect of alcohol on the overall occurrence of seizures in PWE that we completed at the time provided an overall relative risk (RR) meningitis of 3.0 (95% CI 2.33–3.77), which was statistically significant. This is the retrospective longitudinal VENICE data with new information after a new seizure risk factor was identified. Two sub-studies, one of exclusively hospital-based PWE and one cumulating the results of previous publications (reducing the impact of the "file drawer" problem), revealed a greater risk of alcohol-related seizures with an RR of 34 and 20 consecutively. Further in-depth analyses were not possible due to the heterogeneity of the data and insufficient information on alcohol consumption. An American study found a lower odds of alcohol consumption among PWE with isolated unprovoked seizures than suspicions with unprovoked seizures or those with PSU. Respective odds ratios (OR) with 95% CI mentioned were 0.5 (0.3–0.7) and 0.3 (0.1–0.5) (p < 0.0001). Lindsten and colleagues observed that self-reported abuse of alcohol was not related to non-ACS or to diagnosis space. The same conclusion was reached by Van Buren in a study in Seattle with PWE diagnosed with confirmed epilepsy. These studies used PWE control designs and are therefore adequate.

3.1. Research findings on alcohol and seizures. Research seems to indicate a multifaceted relationship between alcohol and epilepsy, characterized by (1) the capacity of alcohol to lower the seizure threshold in humans, (2) lower seizure intoxications occurring at relatively low levels of intoxication, (3) a seizure-free period that occurs during the hangover phase, and (4) the possibility of developing an addiction to alcohol with chronic stimulation. The latter may coincide with the development of alcohol withdrawal seizures, especially in severe alcohol addiction. Among people with epilepsy (PWE) without alcohol problems, however, alcohol does not seem to significantly affect the occurrence pattern of frequent seizures.

## 3.2. Mechanisms of Alcohol-Induced Seizures

The susceptibility to alcohol-induced seizures may be multifaceted, with alcohol increasing blood pressure, inducing fluctuations in receptors associated with susceptibility, neuroinflammation, and BBB leakage, all of which are facilitated to varying degrees during sudden withdrawal or excitation. For example, alcohol can transiently increase sensitivity via sodium channels, followed by chronic reductions in potassium currents including BK and GIRK channels. Alcohol can also lower the threshold for convulsive activity by increasing the excitability of the NMDA receptor and its current level. Withdrawal from alcohol can lead to high levels of norepinephrine in the brain, increase the release of glutamate due to the high level of excitation, reduce the inhibition of GABAA receptors, and neuroinflammation reflect in the release of cytokines and excess beta-endorphin. These factors can compromise the function of the BBB and endothelium in various regions of the central nervous system.

Individuals with epilepsy can experience seizures due to alcohol consumption, and neurons from the limbic structures involved in epileptogenesis are considered to be more sensitive to the proconvulsant effects of alcohol compared to other regions. It is possible that this effect is influenced by the density of ion channels, which may fluctuate between different norepinephrine neurons in different regions of the epileptic brain, leading to an increase in the level of neurons that inhibit the brain, which in turn may lead to seizures. In animal models, resistance to alcohol-induced seizures has been replicated through kindling, showing that ABs are also effective against alcohol-induced seizures and that seizures triggered by alcohol replication also stimulate seizures. BACs can suppress the release of glutamate and thus reduce the excitatory transmission associated with seizures. Another possibility is that ABs may reduce the release of glutamate, which has a higher concentration in the brain of some alcohol-dependent people who have a higher frequency of seizures.

3.2 Alcohol-Induced Seizures

# 4. Recommendations for Alcohol Consumption

The first step is to encourage accurate assessment of the individual's alcohol use by asking these individuals specifically about their alcohol consumption on a regular basis. This then opens the door to provide recommendations and strategies aimed at minimizing the risk of seizure with drinking. For an individual who has seizures, we suggest recommending that these people abstain from drinking alcohol, since this is the only sure way to avoid an alcohol-induced seizure. For an individual who has seizures that have been clearly linked to alcohol consumption, but who does not want to abstain from alcohol, we suggest attempting to build in a "seizure buffer" by optimizing the individual's AED regimen, reducing or abstaining from alcohol while on the itinerary during occasions of heightened risk, and intervening to end the seizure if and when it occurs. Awareness of the risk and pragmatic advice will ideally empower people with epilepsy to make safe and informed decisions regarding their alcohol consumption.

It is estimated that approximately 51% of individuals with epilepsy continue to drink alcohol, and some studies suggest that up to one third of those people have alcohol-related seizures. A recent meta-analysis of the relative risk of seizures with alcohol consumption revealed that people with epilepsy have 3 times the odds of alcohol-related seizures when compared to controls. In order to offset some of the negative consequences or side effects of excessive alcohol use, more recent research has focused on developing practical guidance.

## 4.1. Guidelines for Safe Alcohol Consumption

A. To ensure that an acute effect of alcohol on the body does not lead to status epilepticus or a possible and fatal consequence in some people with epilepsy (i.e., sudden unexplained death in epilepsy, or SUDEP), the following guidelines should be used in any person with active epilepsy: 1. If you wish to drink alcohol, it should be done with a meal or at least in between, never on an empty stomach. 2. Have someone present with you for at least one hour following moderate alcohol intake, to check for safety and to intervene if a seizure occurs. 3. Any person with active epilepsy who develops a hangover, including a mild hangover, should increase their routine maintenance medication by at least 50% the day after drinking.

Even if alcohol consumption is associated with seizure occurrence, individuals with epilepsy - if they choose to drink alcohol - should be provided with certain guidelines in order to ensure that alcohol use is as free of serious health/safety consequences as possible. The following guidelines, contributed by one of the authors with epilepsy, aim to highlight practical recommendations and considerations when establishing safe alcohol use.

## 4.2. Strategies to Minimize Risk of Seizures

It is impossible to totally exclude the risk for an epileptic seizure. Yet these measures are less stigmatizing and give the person with epilepsy more feelings of control over life and lifestyle, including choices in participating in social life and enjoying an alcoholic drink. Therefore, the question is not when preventive medication should be ingested, but rather, what activities are planned (what is the probability that an attack will occur?). Knowledge of individual triggers will help a man with epilepsy to prevent seizures. There are several proactive strategies to minimize the risk. Regular and sufficient sleep, low and regular consumption, avoiding a high concentration of alcohol in the blood and a high speed of alcohol consumption. An example is the avoidance or at least minimizing the risk of suffering from a seizure triggered by alcohol. The aim is to not reduce the risk of seizures per se but for the subjects to work towards minimizing the chances of suffering seizures. Because the speed of elimination of alcohol differs from one person to the other, another topic is whether an individual can predict or correct his/her own behavior to minimize the chances.

Therefore, in the first place, one should drink appropriate amounts of alcohol. However, instead of waiting and counting whether triggering is happening, a simple, possibly more effective method is to avoid the increased probability of an alcohol-trigger. A main message in the response might be: Effects of alcohol can be different, the interaction with medication and the threshold is not predictable. To save a fun night, you should take measures in time, e.g., do not consume alcohol too fast, mix drinking with other activities, eat enough, sleep enough. If you are thirsty after alcohol consumption, also drink water. Some more concrete advice for people with epilepsy which is not under well-controlled conditions could be: Do not drink alcohol in the late evening/night, do not go to bed intoxicated, bring along your medication in case you drift away from home or your plan, make agreements with your partner/friend on the amount of alcohol.

4.2. Strategies to minimize the risk of seizures

# 5. Conclusion and Future Directions

Recommendations for clinical management and treatment include: (i) General practitioners should give advice to people with epilepsy about alcohol in general, and as to when it might start being a problem, during consultations concerning medication reviews or medication changes. During such consultations, general practitioners should consider the co-emergence of anxiety, depression, and drinking as part of the presentation of overload. This overload might be part and parcel of one-off trigger provoking seizures in people whose usual seizure type is unrelated to drinking. The provision of information might take the form of exploring the number of units of alcohol that a person feels they can consume on social occasions so as not to trigger seizures, and pointing out that the increased vulnerability to alcohol in epilepsy can make alcohol an apparent trigger in anyone with epilepsy feeling overloaded. - In parallel, as it has been shown that epilepsy is not understood in isolation from co-morbidities, further investigation of the prescribing practices of general practitioners in the case when people present to them with anxiety, depression, seizures, and alcohol is recommended. - In line with the first recommendation, the provision of information should aim to reduce the psychologizing of blame and shame associated with seizures and should outline the neurobiological basis for alcohol as a trigger. The neurobiology leaflet has started to be used in the Nottingham clinic, funded by a South Yorkshire Brain Tumour Appeal grant, and is available in Chapter 7 to be freely copied and adapted for others to use. It has been a successful communication aid for people with epilepsy in the clinic.

- Whereas general practitioners are informed about alcohol as a risk factor for seizures and are also aware that people with a diagnosis of epilepsy can respond differently to alcohol, this knowledge is not necessarily made operational in their clinical encounters with people with epilepsy. General practitioners suggested that they approach the management of alcohol and epilepsy within their consultations on a case-by-case - combined with a general, typical patient - basis. The research findings presented in this thesis suggest three essential strategies for helping people with epilepsy who report that alcohol consumption has an impact on their seizures.

Alcohol is a well-documented risk factor for epilepsy and seizures. Edged by the gaps in knowledge regarding the impact of alcohol on individuals with epilepsy and the management of alcohol-related epilepsy in clinical settings, my primary recommendations are fundamental to increasing basic information and tools. In conclusion, the following major findings on the impact of alcohol in people with epilepsy and conditions for further research and interventions follow from this thesis.